THE WHITE WITCHES' GRIMOIRE

CHANNELED BY
Sangeeta Kalyan Kaur

With love,
for love,
and through love.
For you, who trusted in
acquiring this book.

I walk hand in hand
with you.

I grant you the power to
find your freedom.

Sangeeta Kalyan Kaur.

Table of Contents

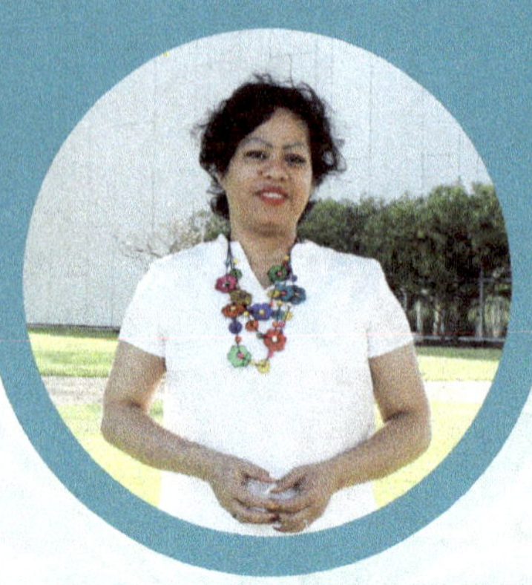

Writer's Note

It's crucial for me to share this information with you before you embark on this journey. I believe it's essential for you to be aware of it before diving into the experience that led you to acquire or choose this book.

The presence, or absence, of the paternal figure in our lives significantly influences our ability to stand up for ourselves, to express our place in the world, to dare to act, and to pursue what we desire. It's the essence of saying, "This is who I am." When this father figure is missing, we often face challenges in defending ourselves, accepting too much because of an overabundance of lunar feminine energy, which makes it difficult for us to set boundaries. Yet, setting boundaries is also an act of self-love and compassion, especially when done in a balanced way.

Photography by Edgar Rafael Garzón Pardo

At times, fear of being hurt can lead us to overcompensate by establishing too many boundaries. However, there are moments when it's necessary to draw the line, especially when someone oversteps their bounds. If not addressed, these unspoken words and actions can later manifest as illness—something that, when examined more deeply, could stem from past-life karmas but also serves as a form of negative karma affecting you in the present.

Not speaking up, not defending yourself, often has its roots in fear. Remember that the Goddess Durga wields not only swords but also flowers and perfumes, and you must be able to draw on both without hesitation.

The absence of feminine power, this masculine aspect of our personality, has long been overshadowed by patriarchy, stripping us of that power. In response, today's women have often swung to the opposite extreme.

We have adopted masculine traits as a defense mechanism against men. But is this truly what we desire? We start mirroring their behaviors, losing touch with our own sensitivity and inner desires. Nowadays, I can choose to have relationships with any man I want, and while society may accept this, I must ask myself—is this truly what I want?

If you can say "yes," that's valid. However, many women today might find themselves saying, "Actually, I'm fine engaging in casual encounters with men." But is that truly what you want? Or is it a form of settling—a defensive stance to avoid being hurt—instead of seeking a deeper connection? The ability to establish boundaries is also closely tied to healing your life and overcoming any abuse or trauma you may have experienced.

Whether it's the experience of abuse, the lack of an apology, or the fact that you may have never expressed your feelings to avoid conflict, all of these unresolved issues can deeply affect you, shaping the life you're living today. Together, through this book, we will begin the journey toward healing.

Although this text primarily focuses on feminine energy, it's equally important to recognize the role of masculine energy. Both men and women possess these energies, and they impact our surroundings in similar ways.

The White Witches' Grimoire

This small manual gathers rituals, purification baths, path-opening practices, liberation from witchcraft, envy, healing, and guidance from angels, archangels, ascended masters, the Holy Spirit, and our ancestors. All the rituals, baths, and advice you find here and wish to perform will be guided by them, granting you the responsibility to ensure no harm is done to anyone. This manual is specifically designed to facilitate your personal liberation and evolution.

What happens if you act against or without the permission of another person? You would be generating significant karma by violating their free will. For this reason, I urge you to carry out each ritual revealed here with the utmost responsibility, ensuring that no one is harmed in the process.

You might wonder, "But what if it's my child, my spouse, my mother, etc.?" It's important to remember that every individual has their own life experience, which must be respected, even if their path is a difficult one. It is our responsibility to accept their journey as they choose to live it, until they decide to change it themselves.

A Very Important Piece of Advice for You Before Starting Any Ritual Found Here

It's crucial that you observe your mind and the beliefs you hold as you approach what is presented here. If you acquired this book believing you are affected by witchcraft, I invite you to pause for a moment, reflect on what your mind is telling you, and review your life's journey.

Why this advice? It's easy to get carried away by the negative messages of the mind, but building a positive life becomes a challenge, especially during times of emotional, physical, mental, or spiritual turbulence—such as when money is tight or you've lost your job.

I want to remind you how the adult mind functions: much like a two-year-old child who is just learning to walk. You cannot leave it unattended because a disaster might occur. Similarly, if you let your mind wander without supervision, it will create a terrifying scenario, leading you to worry about an uncertain future filled with events that often never happen.

Yes, witchcraft exists, but before giving importance to something that likely does not affect you, take a deep breath and ask yourself how relevant you truly are for someone to invest their time in harming you. By withdrawing power from that belief, it ceases to exist.

Remember to observe your mind constantly, and never leave it unsupervised. Guide it toward the life, peace, and harmony you wish to experience in this present moment.

We continue working together. This process doesn't end here; we keep moving forward, stronger than you can imagine. We walk this path together. I give you a warm embrace.

The First Piece of Advice Comes from Archangel Michael

Archangel Michael emphasizes the importance of understanding how life works—your life—in order to avoid making mistakes when trying to save your loved ones. Imagine that life is like a novel, where each actor plays a specific role. Similarly, in this "real life," your loved ones act according to the roles they've chosen or that we've assigned to them. It's not our job to save them, but we can offer them this knowledge as a gift, allowing them to make their own decisions and learn from them. Does this idea resonate with you?

Having said all this, I leave you free to perform the rituals mentioned here, with responsibility, as you open your path and sacred space, seeking only the assistance of beings of light such as the seven archangels, ascended masters, Jesus, and Mary.

Below, I share with you the prayer that you should always use whenever you perform any of the rituals revealed in this book.

Power Prayer for Each Ritual or Bath

In accordance with the will of God and in the name of Jesus Christ, in peace and harmony for myself and the entire world, I, "[Say your name]," at this moment, open a sacred space where I invite the beloved Holy Spirit, the seven archangels, the ascended masters, my ancestors, and my spiritual guides, the Father, and the Mother, to assist me in performing "[mention your ritual or bath you are doing at this moment]." Here, you may mention everything you wish to release or attract into your life, saying: I ask for it in accordance with the will of God, in the name of Jesus Christ, in peace and harmony for myself and the entire world. Thank you, Father, May it be so.

With this prayer, the sacred space is opened, connecting me solely with the beings of light to whom I have asked for help, as guided by the Holy Spirit, for there is no degree of difficulty in miracles. What I have asked for is done, and I request it in this way to ensure that no one is harmed and that, if I am attempting to manifest money, it happens in the most harmonious, appropriate, and liberating way possible. Otherwise, I might manifest the desired amount in a tragic way, such as through a car accident, for example. Or if I am trying to manifest a partner, I ensure they are free of commitments, exclusively for me.

What happens if we don't recite this prayer before every ritual or bath we perform? We would be acting from a place of selfishness, from the ego, which could bring us negative consequences. But this will not be, nor is it, your case, as you are following the guidance provided in this manual. Allow yourself to be guided, and let's continue with your liberation.

Thank you for being here; the spiritual world accompanies you. And the one speaking to you at this very moment is Archangel Michael, the Warrior, who stands by your side today and always. I open the path for all my brothers who will offer their tools to heal your journey.

With affection,
Archangel Michael.

Spiritual Purification Baths

Message from the Herbs

We, the herbs, gather here, filled with pride, to offer you our essence and our spirit. We are deeply proud of you. I, Rue, speak on behalf of my companions, and we want to express our joy in granting you our energy to heal and release all that no longer serves your path—not just yours, but that of your entire lineage.

We have been in service to humanity for millions of years, and our ancient existence grants us the power of salvation and liberation. It fills us with happiness that you have accepted our help and are putting it into practice. When a soul is freed, an entire world is liberated; you have no idea how many souls are released when you choose to free yourself.

This is why we feel such pride when you choose us and allow us to share our energy with you. It is a tremendous joy and a great honor to be at your service. I am the energy of Rue, accompanied by the energy of Rosemary and Sage. We are very happy that you have chosen to heal, not only for yourself but also for your ancestors, your future descendants, your future children, and grandchildren.

We want to reiterate the joy of having you here, liberating yourself and being part of your spiritual growth. We thank our guide for making this connection possible.

Note

These cleansing, healing, and purification baths, as well as the path-opening baths and certain rituals, are equally effective for businesses, whether physical or digital.

Recommendations

For a physical business, once you've performed a cleansing bath, whether at night or in the morning before opening your business, you should conduct the same bath for your establishment. Here, you will sweep and mop your physical business from the back of the establishment toward the entrance, using the bath you prepared beforehand. Remember to recite the power prayer while doing this cleaning, infusing your business with the intention of purification. This protocol can also be applied to your home, and it's recommended to clean your business or house immediately after cleansing yourself.

Imagine you exercised at the gym and took a shower, but then put on the same gym clothes again; it would be contradictory. In the same way, after cleansing yourself, you should also cleanse the space where you spend your time, whether it's your business or your home.

For a digital business, it's sufficient to visualize yourself cleansing your website, online store, social media profiles, etc., after you've cleansed yourself, because, at the end of the day, you are the face of your business, whether it's physical or digital.

I wish you all the success in the world as you perform these baths and rituals, both for yourself and for your businesses, work, or home.

First Bath

This first bath, given by Archangel Gabriel, is designed to help you release any negative energy that has attached itself to you, whether it was sent by someone else or created by yourself. As you know, your mind has the power to generate unnecessary situations that prevent you from seeing the blessings in your life, creating a perception of scarcity in areas such as finances, health, peace, harmony, and more.

Following the prayer protocol presented at the beginning of this book, you will perform this bath for three consecutive days.

Ingredients:

- Bay leaves
- Three garlic cloves
- Peppercorns
- Coffee
- Tobacco
- Water
- New clothing

Procedure:

In 3 liters of water, place all the ingredients and let them boil for 30 minutes. If the water reduces too much, add more water. After the bath, you will wear new clothing, as expected.

Once the bath is prepared and after following the main prayer protocol, bathe as you normally would. At the end, and based on your personal situation and what you need at this moment, proceed to pour the infused water over yourself using a smaller container, saying, for example: "Through you, I release myself from [mention what you wish to be freed from]."

Finish this procedure without drying off completely; allow your skin to absorb what you have just done. Simply place a towel on your head to prevent the water from dripping. If you prefer, lightly pat a towel over your intimate areas, such as your armpits and other parts.

We conclude this procedure by giving thanks to the Father, the Son, and the Holy Spirit, as well as to our ancestors and spiritual guides for their assistance.

Second Cleansing Bath

This is a cleansing bath, designed to remove all negativity from your life, including any witchcraft, if present.

Ingredients:

- White flowers
- Peppercorns
- Garlic
- 3 liters of water

Procedure:

Boil 3 liters of water and add the petals of the white flowers, peppercorns, and garlic. Let it boil for 30 minutes. Once it reaches a tolerable temperature (lukewarm, for example), proceed to bathe as you normally do. After completing your regular bath, take the prepared water (previously strained) and, as you pour it over yourself, say:

"Blessed water, consecrated by the Holy Spirit and my beloved archangels, through you, I release this misfortune that I am experiencing" (describe the specific problems you are facing here).

With this act, declare your liberation from witchcraft, curses, envy, or any negativity affecting you. It's important not to dry yourself immediately afterward; allow your body to absorb the purifying energy of the water. Only dry your intimate areas and place a towel on your hair if desired.

Advice from Archangel Zadkiel

Remember to perform these baths with the responsibility that comes with being an adult, as they are powerful rituals intended for your personal liberation. These baths are meant exclusively for you. If you wish to help a family member or someone important in your life, it would be best to share this book with them, allowing them to undertake their own process of liberation.

I leave you in peace and harmony, and may you receive my blessing in the name of the Father, the Son, and the Holy Spirit.

With affection,
Archangel Zadkiel.

Purification Bath

Ingredients:

- Salt
- Flower Water
- Rue leaves

Procedure:

This bath is simple, so don't overcomplicate it. If, for any reason, you only have salt, that will be sufficient. Following the opening prayer protocol, wet your body and then mix the salt with Flower Water and rue to exfoliate your entire body. Ask the salt to heal and cleanse any misused energy or any heavy sensation you may feel. Performing this bath at night will help you rest deeply, freeing you from energetic burdens.

Message from Archangel Gabriel

Beloved, this is the time to cleanse, purify, and heal, freeing yourself from the chains that bind you. It is crucial to remember that you have left your mind unattended, and if left unsupervised, it can lead you to destruction or elevate you toward success. I am here to enlighten and guide you; I love you, and it is out of love that I protect you. Allow me to guide your steps in the name of Jesus. We continue together, thank you.

With affection,
Archangel Gabriel.

Cleansing with a Bundle of Herbs

Ingredients:

- Rue
- Rosemary
- Sage
- White carnation
- Red carnation

Procedure:

Create a bundle with intention, using the white and red carnations as an offering to your spiritual guides and ancestors. Following the initial prayer protocol, sweep your body from top to bottom with the bundle, never in the opposite direction. Take your time, and when you finish, place the bundle on the ground and rub your bare feet over it, asking for success and financial abundance in alignment with your life experience.

Cleansing with Copal

Copal, a special resin used by various cultures to purify the environment and ward off negative energies, is a powerful element for both personal and home energy cleansing. Use an appropriate container to burn a piece of copal previously designated for you, programming it with your intentions of liberation and purification. Allow the smoke to do its work while you recite your intentions for cleansing, always with care and responsibility.

These procedures, offered with intention and respect, are powerful tools for your spiritual and energetic well-being. Always remember to proceed with responsibility, being mindful of the power of your intentions and the natural elements at your disposal.

Cleansing with Egg or Green Lemon

For this cleansing, you can use a fresh egg, preferably with a brown shell. If you're wondering whether you can use a white or refrigerated egg due to your location, remember that faith is the driving force behind this ritual. Therefore, if you can't find a fresh brown egg, don't worry—use whatever you have on hand, whether it's an egg or a green lemon. Both are equally effective as long as you perform the ritual with faith.

Following the prayer protocol, requesting the assistance of your ancestors, spiritual guides, the beloved Holy Spirit, and the archangels, proceed to pass the egg or green lemon over your body from head to toe while reciting the prayer. If you're using an egg, make sure not to break it; the intention is to rid yourself of negative energies. Immediately place the egg or lemon in a black bag and dispose of it as far away from your home as possible, in a location you don't frequently pass by. This simple ritual of energetic cleansing will leave you feeling a significant change.

Flourishing Baths

Message from Archangel Michael

Remember, in this process of cleansing and healing, you are never alone. We accompany you, holding your hand, ensuring that everything turns out well. I, Michael the Warrior, have raised my sword in your defense and will continue to do so, protecting you like a warrior brother. I will never tire of showing you my love, for I am here for you, helping you bring out your best self. Those who underestimated you will see your triumph, for with me and the Holy Spirit by your side, you are blessed on this journey.

We continue together.

With affection, Archangel Michael.

Using the Flourishing or Road-Opening Bath

After cleansing your energy of all negativity, it's time to perform a Flourishing Bath, also known by many as a Road Opener. This ritual is beneficial both personally and for your business or work.

Flourishing Bath:

Ingredients:

- White rose petals
- Red rose petals
- Cinnamon
- Bay leaves

Procedure:

Boil all the ingredients in 3 liters of water. Bathe following the protocol of the initial prayer, and as you use this mixture, ask for success and flourishing in the aspects of your life you wish to improve, such as spiritual growth, financial prosperity, or success in work or business. This bath should be performed for three consecutive days, preferably wearing a new garment after each session, whether daytime clothing or pajamas for the night. This ritual will help you open paths and attract prosperity and well-being into your life, marking a new beginning filled with blessings and growth.

Second Flourishing Bath

Ingredients:

- Colorful flowers (roses, daisies, or any others you prefer—the important thing is to choose colors you feel connected to)
- Flower Water
- Seven Machos Cologne
- Your favorite perfume
- White sugar
- White vinegar

Recommendation:

This flourishing bath is ideal to perform on the first day of each month.

Procedure:

If you have a bathtub, fill it with warm water and add the bouquet of flowers along with the other ingredients. If you don't have a bathtub, boil water in a pot, turn off the heat, add the ingredients, cover the pot, and let it steep for a few minutes before using. Immerse yourself in this mixture and allow yourself to enjoy the bath for as long as you wish. Avoid drying off immediately so your body can absorb all the energy from the components.

This ritual, shared by Archangel Gabriel, is designed to enhance flourishing in various areas of your life.

Don't be surprised if people around you start noticing a change, asking what you've done to look so radiant. It's your responsibility to respond with the best attitude, allowing others to see the success and flourishing within you.

Sweetening Bath

Ingredients:

- 100% pure coconut oil
- Cinnamon
- White sugar

Procedure:

Mix these three ingredients in a bowl. As you combine them, focus on sweetening your path according to your desires and life experiences. Coconut oil, along with cinnamon and sugar, are powerful attractors of positive energies.

Before bathing, recite the preliminary prayer to invoke protection and guidance. Then, wet your body and begin exfoliating from your face to your feet, asking to attract everything you wish to improve or obtain in your life—be it a new romantic relationship or a more fulfilling job.

These baths are not only designed to cleanse your energy and open pathways to success and prosperity but also to bring sweetness into your life, allowing you to experience more rewarding and love-filled moments.

With affection, Archangel Gabriel.

Rituals for Beginners

Introduction

These rituals, designed for anyone, are short and effective. Remember to use the preliminary prayer provided at the beginning, and keep in mind that faith is crucial in everything you do. Anything done with faith and the initial prayer will be much easier and more effective, as we ask for what rightfully belongs to us without harming anyone or opening doors to energies not aligned with our perfect vibration. These rituals are effective for eliminating illnesses, emotional attachments, limiting beliefs, and attracting the desired job and partner, among others.

What Is an Emotional Attachment?

An emotional attachment occurs when a past hurt continues to affect you, preventing you from moving forward in life. For example, it could be mistreatment by a parent during childhood, being forced to have an abortion in your youth, or growing up in poverty. These emotional attachments are our responsibility to eliminate from the subconscious, as they hinder us from living a full and free life. To address this, we must first become aware of what we carry ancestrally. At the end of this text, you'll find a bonus meditation that you should record on your mobile device to listen to, depending on what you're carrying in your life.

What Is a Limiting Belief?

A limiting belief might be feeling obligated to bear family illnesses, workplace abuses, or toxic relationships inherited from our ancestors. For example, it can manifest as the belief that diabetes or cancer are common in your family, or that they've always been poor. These emotional deficiencies, from birth to the present, limit us from living a full and desired life, influencing the scarcity of money, toxic relationships, and financial limitations. Recognizing and eliminating these ancestral inheritances is crucial for living our own lives. This text is inspired by Archangel Raphael.

Ritual Number One to Eliminate Negative Beliefs or Energies

Ingredients:

- A clove of garlic
- Sea salt
- Paper
- Pencil
- White candle

Procedure:

1. Write on a piece of paper what you wish to eliminate (negative energies, arguments, limiting beliefs, etc.).

2. Insert the paper into the clove of garlic.

3. Take a handful of sea salt and, with a triumphant attitude, raise your arm upward while saying: "I, [your name], release you and let you go; I no longer give you the power to direct my life." Repeat this three times.

4. Bury the garlic and say to Mother Earth: "I give you this energy; please use it for your benefit and the good of all your inhabitants."

5. With the white candle, pass it over your entire body (ensure the candle is not in a glass container) and speak to the energy of the candle, saying: "Hello candle, from this moment you represent my body. Through you, I incorporate [mention what you wish to bring into your life]."

Ritual for Money

It's important to bless your finances, work, and home. Perform this ritual once a week, ideally on the first working day.

Ingredients:

- Ground cinnamon
- White sugar

Procedure:

1. Place a handful of cinnamon and sugar in the palm of your hand.

2. Bring your palms together and, with your eyes closed, recite the preliminary prayer while visualizing a shower of money coming to you.

3. Rubbing your hands with the ingredients, say: "I open myself to economic and professional success."

This ritual is inspired by Archangel Gabriel.

Ritual of Divine Providence

This ritual is performed so that nothing is ever lacking in your home, ensuring food and the payment of bills or rent.

Ingredients:

- White candle
- Rice
- Lentils
- Corn
- Sugar
- White plate

Procedure:

1. Speak to the white candle, acknowledging its existence and welcoming it into your universe.

2. Visualize what you wish to incorporate into your environment while holding the candle between your hands.

3. Place the candle on the white plate and speak to each of the ingredients; for example, to the rice: "As you grow, so does my prosperity."

4. Light the candle and welcome each ingredient, sweetening your ritual.

This ritual is inspired by the angels of abundance.

These rituals are designed to cleanse your energy, open paths to success and prosperity, and attract positivity into your life. May they help you embark on a new beginning filled with blessings and growth.

A Token of Gratitude

Free yourself and soar as high as the eagles. To suffer or not is entirely up to you!

Ancestral Liberation Meditation

This ancestral liberation meditation is a gift for you, beneficial for both women and men, as ancestral energies affect us all equally. Remember, it's your responsibility to record this meditation on your mobile device and listen to it as often as you need.

Close your eyes and allow yourself to be guided by the beloved Holy Spirit, who will offer direction throughout this meditation. Feel the presence of Mother Mary, who comes to help us transcend what we, as humans, have yet to achieve: liberating and acknowledging the adult within us.

With your eyes closed, take a deep breath, holding the air for a moment before releasing it. Feel yourself expelling all that misused energy. With each deep breath, visualize all the accumulated stress in your body dissipating.

Now, focus your attention on any unresolved emotions or conflicts with your parents or ancestors. Connect with these feelings and notice where they resonate in your body. If you feel the need to cry, let it out; tears are a means to free the soul. Don't hold back.

Becoming aware of these emotions and conflicts, place your hand on the area where you feel them and repeat: "I forgive myself, and I forgive you; I release myself, and I release you." Do this three times, affirming both your liberation and theirs.

From your adult self, declare: "Now, as the adult I am, I set you free." Remove your hand and allow yourself to feel the release. Imagine the energetic ties that still bind you to your ancestors. Observe how these bonds, darkened by life's negative experiences, remain attached to you.

To your right, visualize a pair of scissors. Take them with your right hand and, with gratitude and without resentment, say: "I forgive you, and I forgive myself." As you do this, see how the bond is cleansed, returning the energy backward, acknowledging that what you're experiencing doesn't belong to you, as you've been, in some way, living the lives of your parents or ancestors.

Now cut all the energetic ties and set yourself free. Take a deep breath and, only when you're ready, open your eyes. Become aware of your body in this present moment, feeling free and ready to live your life fully, rising like the eagles to the highest heavens.

SECOND PART

Well, we have completed the first part of this book. Now it's time to assess the potential changes by applying the tools and healing messages you've implemented in your life up to this point. Below, you'll find a section where you can write a summary analyzing how you feel in your life after reading this part and applying what you've learned.

It's essential that you put this into practice because today marks your ancestral liberation. What do I mean by "ancestral healing"? The moment has come to leave behind superficial games and rituals. Your "onion moment," as I like to call it, has arrived. This means we're going to dive deep into your complete healing. We'll work on healing your relationships with your mother, your father, your ex-partners, and your ancestors. Are you ready?

Let's get started…

Welcome to the second part of your healing. It's crucial that you've reached this point after analyzing how you did with the first part of this book because now we're fully entering into your freedom—the freedom you've been seeking for years but haven't been able to find. We'll begin by cutting ties with your parents, especially with your mother, which is the connection we still maintain. Even if she's no longer in this plane, the connection continues. It's necessary to work on releasing what binds us to her and, once and for all, stop living her repetitive life story, allowing ourselves the will to live our own story—a story of peace, harmony, abundance, good relationships, fulfilling jobs, great friendships, and wonderful children, including those we'd like to have.

For this journey, we'll delve once again into analyzing how our history has been in areas like love, money, friendships, and more.

Use the pages below to jot down notes on these topics. This way, when we proceed with the healing, you can refer back to them and see how you've freed yourself and progressed in your life. From here on, you'll find three lined pages where you can write and reflect on the subjects we'll be working on. Use them to contemplate and document your thoughts and feelings about the themes discussed in this chapter.

Assuming you already have the topics you want to work on in your life, let's begin by discussing pains in your body. We won't delve too deeply because the idea is to make you aware, guiding you by the hand, recognizing where your possible limitations come from so you can bring them to emotional, spiritual, and physical healing. The right side of the body is associated with the masculine aspect, which means that if you have any pain in that part of your body, it may be linked to success in your life, as success is granted by the father.

Meanwhile, the left side is related to the feminine, connected to emotional conflicts. When these polarities are not balanced in our lives, it's of great importance to harmonize these energies by healing and releasing any conflict we have with our parents, thereby healing and balancing our feminine and masculine energy. For this work, we will carry out several exercises that will help us release. I will share with you some letters that personally helped me a lot in healing the masculine and feminine sides by writing these letters to my parents.

Don't worry; you don't have to give these letters to your parents or anyone else to whom they might apply, and they don't even have to be in this plane of existence. If your parents have already passed away, you should still do this release. And if you were fortunate enough not to have known either of them, you should do it all the same, and even more so. Conversely, if you were raised by a relative, grandparents, or were adopted, besides doing this letter or healing with your parents, you should also do it with these figures. In other words, you will perform double healing.

Below, I share some letters that will help you free yourself from attachments to your parents, ancestors, and others.

Letter of Forgiveness to the Father Who Abandoned You

Dear Father,

I, "your name," am writing to you at this moment because I've realized that much of what I've suffered has been due to the abandonment you subjected me to by leaving me alone since my birth. I acknowledge that I always missed you greatly, that your absence was very painful for me, and that I longed for you immensely. As a consequence, I always sought a man in my life who would give me what you never did. How ironic, because what I always received from those partners was abandonment. Today, I realize why that happened. Today, I understand that I never overcame your abandonment and that with every partner I met along the way, it was always you I was seeking.

That's why they always ended up abandoning me. But today, I am an adult who is taking responsibility for my healing. Today, I realize that if you abandoned me, it's probably because you also experienced abandonment from your own father. Therefore, I cannot ask you for anything or blame you for anything, since you weren't capable of giving me what you didn't have to give. That is why today, at this moment, from the depths of my heart and with all my love, I forgive you, I release you, and I set you free. I grant you your freedom now, knowing that at some point in our spiritual journey, we will meet again, and that encounter will be one of healing, filled with love and respect. Father, I love you. Despite everything, I let you go, I wish you happiness, and I remain open to our reunion. Wherever you are, receive my love, my forgiveness, and continue in peace. I love you.

This is the letter that I share with you with all my love. You can use this sample letter for every person in your life whom you wish to forgive, release, and set free—anyone related to your upbringing or someone from whom you learned something that you now realize has been controlling your life repeatedly. Enough of living a mediocre life; it's time to embrace living life in fullness as we deserve. I ask you to continue blessing your path. We continue healing together through this writing granted by Archangel Raphael.

Letter of Forgiveness to Your Parents

Dear Father and Mother,

I, "your name," am writing to you at this moment because I've realized that much of what I've suffered has been due to the abandonment you caused me by leaving me alone to dedicate so much time to work, with the total responsibility of caring for my siblings since my birth. Your abandonment became evident; I acknowledge that I always greatly missed your company and your love, but it was always the opposite. Your absence was very painful for me; I missed you both tremendously. As a consequence, I always sought a man in my life who would give me what you never gave me. How ironic, because what I always received from those partners, friends, and bosses was abandonment.

Today, I realize why that happened. Today, I understand that I never overcame your abandonment and that the partners and people I related to along the way—in each of them, it was always you I was seeking. That's why they always ended up abandoning me. But today, I am an adult who is taking responsibility for my healing. Today, I realize that your situation wasn't a real abandonment—that you only went out to work—and perhaps you, too, experienced similar abandonment from your parents. Therefore, I cannot ask you for anything or blame you for anything, since you weren't capable of giving me what you didn't have to give. That is why today, at this moment, from the depths of my heart and with all my love, I forgive you, I release you, and I set you free. I grant you your freedom and return all the negative lessons learned, all the deficiencies. Now, knowing that at some point in our history there will be no record of anything I might have inherited or learned, from this moment spiritually, emotionally, and physically, everything is forgiven and released. No record remains. I let you go; continue on your path just as I will continue on mine. I wish you happiness. Receive my love, my forgiveness, and continue in peace and love. I love you.

Letter of Release with Ancestresses

In the divine presence and with God's permission, I now release all that no longer serves me—all the false beliefs that limit me. I release attachments and beliefs that do not contribute to my spiritual and personal growth. With love and gratitude, I thank my ancestors for all they have given me and release any burdens that have been passed down to me. I lovingly let go of fears and karmic contracts that no longer serve me. I free myself from scarcity programming and open my heart to abundance. I declare that I deserve to live a life full of love and prosperity. I release poverty, lack, violence, and illness. My being fills with love and divine light, and I allow this energy to flow through me to heal any aspect of myself that needs it. I renounce the need to always be right and release the belief that I don't deserve to put myself first. I appreciate life in all its forms and live in constant gratitude. I make a contract with my soul to love myself in this life and others, to live in continuous expansion and growth. I accept that I am a being worthy of love, joy, and success in all areas of my life.

After writing each letter, take a moment of reflection. You may feel emotionally wounded—this is entirely normal, especially when dealing with the abandonment of a father. It doesn't necessarily have to be abandonment in the literal sense; perhaps your father, mother, or anyone involved in your upbringing simply had to leave to work, but your subconscious perceived it as abandonment. That's where it all begins. You can use each letter for any situation you wish to forgive or release in your life. Of course, this letter can also help you forgive ex-partners. I've provided these letters as examples because I know that when you're in this healing process, you might feel blocked and not know how to start a forgiveness letter. Please adapt each of these letters to your life situation.

When you write each of these letters to release and heal, please deeply analyze your life story, taking your ancestors into account. With your mother lies the deepest bond that ties us back more than seven generations—this includes grandmothers, great-grandmothers, great-great-grandmothers, and beyond. What do I mean by this? Remember that our ancestors experienced violations, physical, mental, and emotional abuses, economic hardship, machismo, and more. These were commonplace in their times. If you've gone through something similar in this life—perhaps not as profound or maybe so—only you know your life story. Also, recall that in those times, alcoholism and domestic violence were very common in marriages.

This part is entirely personal. Healing your relationship with your mother can be done through the letters of forgiveness and release. Additionally, we will be doing liberation exercises with her as well. Here, I'd like to share a deep meditation where we will cut all ties with her. This doesn't mean you'll stop seeing her or become her enemy; it works on an energetic level. Physically, if your mother is still alive, you'll be able to have a better relationship with her. You'll learn to love her, respect her, and understand that she couldn't give you what she didn't have herself. I share with you the healing meditation with her.

You should record this meditation in your own voice on your device and listen to it for at least 21 days, or as long as you wish, until you achieve emotional forgiveness. Listen to it every morning and every night before sleeping. With that said, let's proceed to the meditation.

Bond Healing Meditation

Find a comfortable place; you can do this sitting or lying down—whichever is more comfortable for you. In this healing process, it doesn't matter if you fall asleep while listening to the meditation, but never perform it while driving.

Close your eyes and focus on your breathing—slowly and deeply—inhaling through your nose and exhaling through your mouth. Very good. Mentally count down from 10 to 1, and when you reach 1, you'll find yourself in a sphere of white light—a healing light. This space will fill you with peace, harmony, and happiness, because you will finally find freedom from all the deficiencies you've experienced since the moment of your birth. Very good. Enjoy this moment. Stay there, savoring that peace; focus on your breathing. The more you breathe, the more you release, gradually becoming aware of a tube of light entering through the crown of your head, illuminating your entire being and cleansing all the energy that's been embedded there since birth.

In this spiritual space, open your inner vision and see that everything is white, almost transparent. You'll notice a white silhouette approaching you, getting closer with each moment. This fills you with joy because you're about to encounter your freedom—you are about to receive your liberation with love, for love, and to live with the love you deserve. The silhouette draws nearer and nearer. Mentally count from three to one, and now she is right in front of you. She is the most important person in your life: your mother. I want you to visualize how you are energetically connected to her. You'll realize that you're still linked, primarily through the umbilical cord. Then there's a connection from the heart, and emotional ties as well. Every painful emotion you've experienced in this life has a connection with her. I want you to see the cords extending from your body and connecting to her at this moment.

Make visual contact with her and observe her reaction upon seeing you. Whatever her response may be, say these words:

"Mom, I come to you at this moment in my adult life because I have taken responsibility for my healing. I no longer blame you for anything I've had to experience; now I hold myself accountable for everything I've lived through. I can't blame you for not giving me what you didn't receive in your own life. I now understand that your life wasn't easy either, and therefore you couldn't give me what you didn't have. You couldn't treat me differently; you couldn't give me the love you were supposed to because love was the most unfamiliar thing you experienced in your life. My dear mother, today, with love and for love, I release you, I forgive you, and I forgive myself for blaming you for something you're not guilty of. Accept my forgiveness; accept that I return to you everything I learned from you, all that I shared with you over these years of my life. I give it back to you because it belongs to you. I've learned that I must take responsibility for my healing and liberation by following my own path. That's why I've come at this moment—to free myself from you, to let you go, to forgive you and myself, to liberate myself and set you free. This doesn't mean I'll stop loving and respecting you; on the contrary, I do this out of love—for love of you, for love of me, and for the love we both deserve that's coming our way as a result of this healing meditation."

Now observe her reaction to these words. Take a deep breath and embrace her deeply. When you're ready, let her go and take a step back. To your left, a suitcase appears containing some tools, and among them is a pair of scissors. I want you to take those scissors and start cutting all the ties, beginning with the umbilical cord. You'll notice that as you cut each of the cords, they begin to fade and she starts to move away from you. Cut each of the ties that link you to her at this moment. Count down from five to one, and when you reach one, she will have disappeared, leaving you with a sensation of peace, love, and healing. You feel freedom.

Now that she has departed of her own will after you've cut the cords, remain there with your eyes closed, enjoying the healing we've just completed. Take a deep breath and refocus on your peace and your breathing. Gradually, start returning to your body. Become aware of your physical presence. When you're ready, return to the present moment in which you're conducting this meditation.

This was the healing meditation to release your bond with your mother. You can apply it in the same way with your father or any other significant relationship in your life. I hope it has been a great help in your healing journey at this moment. Above all, it brings me immense satisfaction to know that you have undertaken this practice.

Reflect and respond to the following questions:
How did you feel during the meditation?

Describe the emotions and sensations you experienced while engaging in the meditation.

Visualization of the Silhouette
How did you visualize the person with whom you

healed the bond? Describe their appearance and any details that caught your attention.

Emotional Connection

What emotions arose when you visualized the energetic cords connecting you to that person?

Words of Release

How did you feel when expressing words of release and forgiveness? Did you notice any change in your energy?

Reaction of the Person

How did you visualize the reaction of the person (your mother, father, etc.) upon receiving your words? Describe any significant details.

Cutting Energetic Ties

How did you feel when cutting the energetic ties? Was there any resistance, or was it a smooth process?

Feeling of Freedom

After the person disappeared and you were left in peace, what changes did you notice in your body and mind? Describe the sensation of freedom you experienced.

Let's move on to a series of exercises that can help you, and I want to share them because, personally, they were exercises that helped me reach the level I'm at now. I've healed much of what I've gone through in my life and have overcome many things. But without a doubt, freeing myself ancestrally and breaking ties has helped me achieve success in my personal life. That's why I don't want to keep anything to myself that hasn't helped me improve. So I'm sharing a series of exercises you can do.

Exercise Number 1

If your mother and father are no longer with you in this world, or they're in another country, or you never knew them, we know that, in some way, the bonds with them reside within us. To release them, we'll buy a bouquet of white lilies and place it in a vase with water. If you have a photograph or their names, place it in front of the flowers while saying these words:

If you're doing this for your father, say:

"Dad, I offer you these flowers as an offering and a sign of my love and forgiveness. I wish that wherever you are, you are happy and filled with peace, love, and freedom, because that's what I desire for you with all my love. May whatever you're experiencing be lived in happiness and fullness, in peace, in love, with all the love that surrounds you, and that one day we'll enjoy together."

Then, if possible, light a white candle for him.

This is an excellent exercise in forgiveness. You can apply this same exercise with your mother or any other situation or person with whom you want to heal bonds. Again, it also works to release ex-partners, whether they are still in this world or not, or far from you.

Exercise Number 2

In this simple yet highly effective exercise for purification and liberation, I'd like to share the following: while showering, visualize a rainbow emerging from the water that is purifying and cleansing you. As the water flows over you, ask it to help you heal—that just as it cleanses your physical body, it also frees you from the invisible, from everything emotionally embedded within you: all the pain, frustration, sadness, and feelings of lack. Incorporate everything you know from your life story, and you'll feel lighter and freer after each shower. You can perform this ritual as often as you wish until you reach a point where you no longer need it. I hope you give it a try.

Exercise Number 3

Every time you clean your house—whether washing dishes or mopping the floor—make a point to repeat these magical words. For example, while washing dishes, say: "As I clean this plate, I cleanse my soul, my body, my spirit of all karmic ties with my surroundings." Again, apply this to your life story and anything you wish to break ties with. Incorporate it into each of your daily activities until you realize that once you're thoroughly cleansed, you won't need it anymore. It can take as much time as you desire. Remember, this is a play on words that will help you heal. You can also apply it when managing your finances. For example, when you're paying at the supermarket or settling a bill, say: "Through this payment, I settle any karmic debt I have with…" and once again, relate it to your life experience.

I hope that what you've read so far in this second part of the book, "The White Witches' Cookbook," is of great help to you.

Now we move on to another level: freeing ourselves from ex-partners. This part is also very important because it's another aspect that keeps us stagnant. We're all someone's ex, and by being someone's ex, we may continue to carry the energy of that person, even if they're no longer in this realm or many years have passed without communication. How do I know this? Throughout my experience as a therapist, medium, and channeler, I've encountered numerous women aged 57, 65, even 77 who had a youthful love, and during mediumship or hypnosis sessions, this past love appears. It turns out that, without them mentioning that relationship to me, in many cases, that energy is still with them, preventing them from fully realizing themselves as wives to their current partners. I'm talking about 55 or 57 years of marriage to their current spouse. That's why it's crucial to free ourselves from ex-partners. It doesn't matter—I'll repeat it again—whether this individual is in this realm or not, whether you're aware of their existence; you need to free yourself not so that this person can live in peace, but because you deserve to live a perfect, free life, to live your own life story.

In this stage of liberation, I recommend applying the previous exercises, starting with the forgiveness letter. It's time to stop letting yourself be manipulated by energies that aren't yours; it's time for you to live your own life story. It's time to leave the past behind and become conscious of your present, because the past has nothing new to tell you. On the other hand, if you focus on building your present, I assure you that your future will be much better. Focus on yourself, help yourself, and forget about that useless past where you weren't valued or given your place.

At this moment, we won't delve much further because the exercises have already been provided, and you can continue using the same ones, as forgiveness and liberation also apply here. But later on, we will perform two definitive healings that will lead you to successful liberation, where you will become a different person—I assure you, I guarantee it. If you are following everything you've read to the letter, there will surely be a before and after reading this book—I guarantee it. So, start applying the forgiveness letter with each of your ex-partners.

With nothing more to add, we're ready to evaluate everything we've learned in this healing section.

Impact on Your Life

How do you believe these exercises have impacted your life and emotional healing?

PART

THREE

In this third part of the book, we will experience a profound womb healing. I would like to explain why it's important to undergo deep healing of the womb. Of course, we will also conduct an ancestral healing process for men. All of the above is interconnected in some way; that is why these are the most crucial aspects to heal energetically, to liberate ourselves, and once and for all, stop being manipulated by the energies of the family environment, the family tree, or whatever you prefer to call it.

If you analyze it carefully, all of this is connected to what we've been discussing in this book. That's why I left this type of healing for the end. Although the most important part is still to come, and we'll get to that at the very end of the book. You'll soon find out who the most important person we'll be healing is. But first, we need to disentangle everything we've been reading up to this point. How is an energetically ill womb related to your life? Besides everything you've read so far, if you have projects that don't materialize no matter how hard you try, if you're financially stagnant and your money doesn't stretch, if you're in abusive, unfaithful, aggressive, alcoholic, or chauvinistic relationships, if you experience painful menstruation, mood swings, bloating… All of this is linked to what we've discussed up to now, but it originates from the ancestral, past lives, and karmic energy.

For the gentlemen, I will also include ancestral healing, because they too are affected by everything we've discussed so far. In some part of their past lives, they were also women and are dragging these issues along. So, gentlemen, you're not exempt from all of this either.

Here, we will do a series of exercises that will help us to free ourselves deeply.

Let's begin this healing journey:

The only thing awaiting you is healing—feeling better and freeing yourself from everything. Make yourselves comfortable; you can start closing your eyes. We are about to embark on your healing journey.

The first exercise we will do is to open sacred spaces. So, say with me, each of you using your own name:

"I, [your name], here and now, in this space where I find myself today [current date and year], accept and acknowledge that I am in my body. I, [your name], inhabit my body. Once again, I, [your name], from here where I am, affirm and recognize that I am in my body. I am here, now."

Gently pat your heart and say: "I am present here; I exist, I exist. I am [your name], and I exist."

Take a deep breath, acknowledging your presence. Now, let's open the sacred space according to God's will, in the name of Jesus Christ, in peace and harmony for myself and for everyone. I, [your name], open this sacred space, inviting the Father, the Son, and the Holy Spirit, my ancestors, and my spiritual guides to guide me in this beautiful healing process for me now. Thank you, Father. Thank you, Son. Thank you, Holy Spirit. Thank you to all the wonderful light beings that accompany me, the ascended masters, the seven archangels, and the angels who accompany them to assist me. Thank you, thank you, thank you. It is done.

Now, open your eyes.

This is the beginning of a powerful journey into healing and liberation. We'll continue with exercises that will guide you through this transformative process.

Why Is It Important to Cleanse Yourself?

It's important that we cleanse ourselves because, as we already know, we carry countless burdens from our ancestors: economic scarcity, abortions, alcoholism, addictions that occurred in our family, whether known or unknown to us. These patterns have been passed down through generations—abortion, domestic violence, and other traumas have existed for thousands of years, even though we may not have been consciously aware of them. And if we are here today, it's because, in some way, we have accepted the mission to heal our lineage.

If we analyze our lives, we might notice that we don't receive approval for what we're seeking—whether it's a loan, government assistance, a job, or any other opportunity. This lack of approval leaves us stuck, as do relationships that aren't suitable for us—whether it's a romantic partner, a friend, or sometimes, when we help others excessively without understanding why. Sometimes, we're there for everyone else but fail to be there for ourselves.

People, especially in relationships, often subject us to abusive behavior, disrespect, and even insults, and yet, we stay. We get pushed, we're told countless hurtful words, and we remain. This happens because we don't know how to value ourselves, and it's not our fault. Nor is it anyone else's fault; it's because we've accepted to follow that pattern, believing in the idea that "this is my cross, it's the one I must bear." No, it shouldn't be that way. This mentality that "if there's enough for one, there's enough for eight" is a belief from our ancestors, but it doesn't have to be our reality.

That's why, in this deep healing process, we begin by recognizing our existence and acknowledging that we bring our own life experience. It's time to say enough to following that ancestral lineage that keeps us stuck over and over again. It's time to break those ties that no longer serve us now, in this moment.

This meditation is already prepared; you just need to record it and listen to it with headphones.

Healing Meditation

I invite you to close your eyes for a moment, and let's analyze our lives from the moment we came into existence. How was the birth when you were born? Was it a cesarean? Was it a natural birth? How were you received? Let's journey back to that moment. Take three deep breaths, and as you travel back in time, you will find yourself in that significant moment in your life. You'll realize that from that moment, connections were formed from all your lineages, both from your father's side and your mother's. It doesn't matter if you didn't know your father; his legacy is still within you. But don't worry, this is why you're here—to cut those ties once and for all.

Believe deeply, and as you go back in time, you're getting closer to that moment. Now, you can visualize your mother in labor. You're there, only as an observer, without connecting emotionally. In this moment, you will be able to witness what each person was saying at the time of your birth and connect these words with how they have impacted your life now because every detail counts, everything matters. Now, you are capable of hearing everything being said in that moment. I want you to see where in your body those words, those emotions, have settled. Place your physical hand on the part of your body where you feel those emotions, those words.

As you are there, as a spiritual being, you are powerful, you are a healer, because you are now the adult who knows that this child grew up despite the words and experiences at the moment of birth. Now, approach that baby and place your hand where those words and emotions became embedded. Surround that baby with a violet light, a light of transmutation and liberation.

That baby now transforms into a white light. Take three deep breaths. You see how those emotions have disappeared. Now, replace that emotion with an emerald green light. Again, place your right hand where those emotions once were, and let that emerald green light replace every emotion in the baby's little body. Watch as this baby now becomes a happy, healed, and liberated child.

Take a deep breath. Now, look around. Open your spiritual vision and observe how the environment has completely changed. Now, that child is happy, and the environment with those people has transformed; everyone is celebrating your rebirth. I call it rebirth because you've lived through many incarnations, but it's in this one that you free yourself and become aware of who you are. You recognize yourself, you exist, you know that you carry your own path, and you are free from all ancestral scarcity. Now, in this moment, you recognize that you are free, that you exist, and that you have your own life story.

Let's return, and I want you to fill that place where you are with light. I want you to fill it entirely with white light.

And now, when everything is illuminated, bring your hands to your heart, placing your right hand over your left. And now, every time you recall this moment or whenever you need peace, you will remember that you are peace, that you are presence, that you have your own light, your own path. By bringing your hands to your heart, you will acknowledge and remember this; you will be able to connect with yourself at this moment, here and now, in this life. Because you are you, because I am me, because I am, I am, I exist, I exist, I exist, and your name, I "[your name]" exist and have my own story, my own path, and in my story and my path, there is only blessing, freedom, love, and abundance in my life. Thank you.

Now, slowly begin to recognize your body, start coming back, feeling your body. When you feel at peace, you can start opening your eyes.

As you might have realized up to this point, healing our birth is crucial, as this is where our life journey begins according to our life plan and family tree. If you don't set a limit and liberate yourself from this history, you will keep running around in circles like a little mouse in a wheel.

Now, let's move on to the next exercise, for which I genuinely hope that by the end of this book, you have become a transformed person. I hope you have applied everything I have channeled with such dedication for you in this little book.

Second Exercise

You have now realized that there is so much we need to heal and release, and that we have been absurdly guided by our ancestral lineage in this life. I believe it's time to stop thinking that way. It's not that we are consciously thinking about it 24 hours a day, seven days a week; it's simply that we are on autopilot, not even needing to think or connect anymore, just like our breathing. We don't have to remind ourselves to breathe; we do it automatically.

So now, we are going to do a deprogramming exercise focused on money. We have already acknowledged our presence, we have recognized that we exist here and now, and we have accepted that we deserve our own life experience. Therefore, we will now recognize that we are worthy of financial stability. We are aware that money is not lacking, but when we have it, something always happens, and the money slips away.

That's why we will do this deprogramming for money, but you can apply it to any area of your life. Imagine yourself inside a bubble of yellow light, somewhere between golden and orange, similar to the ray of Archangel Uriel. Take a deep breath. You are in that golden-orange bubble, and within it, you will notice a tube extending from your navel down to Mother Earth. At this moment, a ray of light begins to enter through the crown of your head, and another connects with your feet. Both are cleansing and freeing your energy. All stagnation in your life, all the darkness, will start to flow out through that tube connecting with Mother Earth. You will notice it leaving.

Allow this to happen, and at this moment, start to mentally affirm, "I release everything." I release this illness, I release my negative beliefs about money, I release all the abortions that have taken place in my family line, I release all the violence in my family, I release catastrophic deaths, I release it all. Begin to name everything: alcoholism, addictions. Why? Because as you free yourself, you are also freeing your children, grandchildren, and great-grandchildren. It's time to stop going around in circles like a mouse trapped in a wheel. We are liberating ourselves from everything. See how all that darkness leaves and is absorbed by Mother Earth, while what enters your body is pure, crystalline light.

Allow this light to enter, healing and freeing you. Say to yourself mentally: "I, [your name], heal and release. I heal and release. I heal and release."

It is not true that I lack anything because my Father is with me. It is not true that I lack money. It is not true that I lack good relationships, friendships, or a partner. It is not true that I lack anything, for my Father exists for me, and I exist for Him. Father-Mother God, repeat: "Father-Mother God, today I recognize that you exist for me and that I exist for you, and that you are here to give me everything I desire." Father-Mother God, today I recognize that you exist; today I recognize that I exist for you and that you exist for me to provide everything I deserve. Father and Mother God, today I recognize that you exist and that I exist for you, and that you exist to give me everything I desire.

What Do You Desire?

Speak to the Father-Mother God about what you desire: "I desire health, I desire financial abundance,

I desire to be approved in this situation." Specify your exact situation. Name what it is that you wish for—whether it's approval for a loan, a check, or anything else you desire to be granted.

Today, I acknowledge that my Father-Mother God exists for me and gives me everything I desire. Thank you, Father. Thank you, Son. Thank you, Holy Spirit. I wrap myself in the flame of abundance from Archangel Uriel. I wrap myself in the flame of abundance from Archangel Uriel. I wrap myself in the flame of abundance from Archangel Uriel. Archangel Uriel accompanies me, Archangel Uriel opens the way for financial abundance, for abundance in all aspects of my life.

I exist for Archangel Uriel, and Archangel Uriel exists for me. Archangel Uriel provides me with everything I desire. Thank you, Archangel Uriel, for accompanying me, for freeing me. Thank you. Stretch out as if you've just woken up, raise your hands, and in a gesture of triumph, shout three times: "I am triumph."

Thank you for this beautiful healing.

Exercise of Self-Recognition and Forgiveness with Archangel Gabriel

Standing in front of a mirror, look yourself in the eyes. Place your right hand on your heart and say: "I am [your name], I am here and now, I recognize that I am present. I acknowledge my life, I acknowledge my existence, I recognize that God is within me, I recognize that God exists for me, bringing me peace, harmony, and forgiveness. Now, I forgive myself for who I have been. I embrace my past, I release it with love, for love, and in love. In the name of the Father, the Son, and the Holy Spirit, God is within me. Now, I accept my new version, where I walk hand in hand with who I am, the one I choose to be now. I am [your full name] here and now, walking hand in hand with [your name]. Thank you, Father. Thank you, Son. Thank you, Holy Spirit. Thank you, Father."

Archangel Gabriel bows before you, recognizing the essence of the Father within you. Thank you, Archangel Gabriel.

We conclude this healing with a powerful cleansing bath. This bath is to be taken once you have completed the previous exercises.

Impact on Your Life

How do you believe the exercises and meditations from this section have impacted your life and emotional healing?

Commitments and Actions

What actions and commitments are you willing to take to maintain this healing in your daily life?

Welcome to the Second Part of the Third Healing Section of this Book

In this section, you will finally free yourself completely through the exercises we will perform. We will continue to heal, liberate, and forgive ourselves through exercises specially channeled for you, to support your healing, liberation, and forgiveness.

We will heal ancestral debts and burdens, release ourselves, and integrate everything we deserve. We are certain that we deserve these blessings, and with that, we will bring this chapter to a close.

As a first step, close your eyes and ask yourself: with whom do I feel indebted? Perhaps you feel indebted to your mother or another situation. Now, I offer you a spiritual debt repayment exercise.

For example, if you feel indebted to your mother, ask her how much you believe you should pay to settle the debt you have with her. Let her give you a figure; it doesn't matter if she asks for millions and you don't have them. Remember, this is purely spiritual.

Primarily, we are in debt to ourselves. I'm in debt for allowing myself to be mistreated, for allowing others to take advantage of me, for not valuing myself enough, for choosing a mediocre life, or for picking a partner who doesn't complement me and never will.

Since we are all someone's ex, think about all those past relationships where you allowed yourself to be manipulated until you reached your current partner. When you're ready, take a deep breath and continue reading.

Forgiveness and Debt Payment Exercise

Write down the names of the people you want to forgive. If there's more than one and you remember their names, write each one down, for example:

"Juan Perez, I forgive you for: (Here, you'll write everything you forgive that person for.)"

Do this for the entire list of people you wish to forgive or with whom you feel indebted. Once you've finished, fold the paper into four parts, hold it close to your mouth, and say, "I forgive you, I forgive myself," three times. Then burn the paper and dispose of the ashes in your bathroom sink.

For the second part, on a spiritual level, ask each person what amount they would consider enough to clear the debt. For example, if Juan Perez is your ex and his presence still bothers you, and you want him to leave you alone, ask him on a spiritual level what amount he desires to be at peace with you.

The act of repayment is as follows:

Print out a blank check from the internet, write the desired amount that this person mentioned, and perform the act of giving it to them so they will leave you in peace. As simple as this act may be, it allows you to release debts you have with certain people.

Prayer of Archangel Raphael

Archangel Raphael offers us a beautiful prayer:

"I, (your name), declare that I exist. I inhabit this body. I am here and now, fulfilling the will of God. I accept God within my body, I exist for God, and God exists for me. God exists to give me everything I desire, and I exist to offer what He desires from me. I desire my healing and liberation. I am here. I am God in action here."

Visualize a violet light, like a tube of light coming from the universe, and a white light tube of refined energy from Mother Earth. These two tubes connect with each other, cleansing your body with both energies—one flows towards the universe and the other towards Mother Earth. At this moment, there are molecules of light surrounding your body. The stagnant energy from your ancestors and past lives is being transformed into light, peace, love, and harmony throughout your being.

Allow this energy to cleanse your bodies: your light body, your physical body, your mental body, your emotional body, and your Christic body—all of your bodies.

Now, mentally, if you wish, say: "I release and let go of everything that no longer vibrates with my energy, I let it go in love and for love. Forgive me, I forgive you. Thank you."

Integration Work with Archangel Raphael

Archangel Raphael remains very present in this deep healing process and offers us a second integration exercise for everything we wish to manifest: Take a piece of paper and a pencil and write down everything you deserve, everything you want to manifest in your life. Now, place your hands on your heart and become aware of the light you are, shining from your heart with golden sparkles. Take a deep breath, and when you feel ready, bring the paper with everything you deserve to your heart. I want you to visualize yourself in a golden bubble, and outside this bubble is everything you want to integrate into your life. At this moment, connect with your deep and gentle breathing.

Visualize everything you wish to integrate into your life outside your bubble of energy. Keep breathing. You are preparing to bring in everything you deserve. Breathe deeply and gently while visualizing with peace, love, joy, and gratitude that all those things outside your bubble are eager to become part of your life. Begin to direct those emotions towards them, inhaling gratitude and exhaling it, giving it to what's outside. Inhale gratitude, thankful for all you desire because it's waiting to be part of you. Exhale that gratitude and watch as everything starts coming closer to your energetic bubble.

Continue to breathe in gratitude and exhale it. Everything you desire is getting closer, and you know it's almost within reach. Keep breathing. Start visualizing how it begins to rain money, how the environment feels filled with joy, gratitude, grace, peace, and harmony, because everything you want to integrate into your life is now drawing closer, nearly entering.

Now, visualize a tube emerging from your navel, heart, third eye, and sexual center. This tube extends beyond your bubble, and with each breath, everything you wish to manifest in your life starts to integrate into your body and energy. Take a deep breath, and with every inhale, it enters. You breathe in gratitude and exhale gratitude, peace, joy, and love, allowing it to fill your energy with all that you desire. Through these tubes of light, everything you wish for flows in.

Your energy is now completely filled with everything you desire. Visualize yourself and feel the peace and harmony that comes with knowing that now you have everything. It is not true that you lack anything. Now, slowly become aware of your body, here and now. Stay in peace, love, and harmony. When you're ready, open your eyes.

Reminder: It is your responsibility to record this practice and listen to it for as long as you feel necessary.

Womb Healing

Archangel Raphael, deeply present at this moment, offers us a quick, profound, and specific womb healing. He wants to get straight to the point, so let's proceed. As always, it's your responsibility to carry out each of the exercises you've read in this book. Let's begin the healing.

But before we start, I'd like to explain why womb healing is important after all the work we've been doing in this book. First and foremost, it's to detoxify your body, as a woman, from everything you've received through experiences in this life and past lives. It's also crucial to understand that by undergoing a womb healing like the one we're about to do, you are also releasing and healing your female ancestors, your present self, and your future daughters, granddaughters, and great-granddaughters. At the same time, you're affirming all the hard work you've bravely done, integrating all the knowledge shared in this book.

This is the cherry on top; enjoy it, you deserve it.

Womb Healing Steam Bath

Ingredients:

- Rosemary
- Rue
- Chamomile

Instructions for Use:

Boil all the herbs for 30 minutes. Once ready, let the mixture cool down and pour it into a container where you can sit and receive the steam that this blend offers. Sit there for about 15 minutes. Don't forget to open your sacred space with the prayer we've been working on throughout this book. Intentionally set your purpose for this steam bath, confirming that all the work you have done is acknowledged and valued for your great growth. As you sit there, close your eyes and visualize that everything has been healed, released, and forgiven. You know your life story best, and who better than you to put into your own words everything you are healing through this womb healing.

Prepare yourself to experience the freedom of being you and your true essence. Thank you, Father.

"I return your freedom to you, my beloved brother. We never tire of helping you in the spiritual realm; we are always by your side at every moment. No matter what is happening, we are here to assist you in any circumstance in your life. Never doubt that you are alone because you are not. This life experience you are living is in the company of your archangels, your angels, your spiritual guides, the beloved Father-Mother God, and the Holy Spirit who always accompanies you and holds your hand. It has been an immense pleasure to accompany you through the reading of this book of healing, liberation, and forgiveness. We continue walking together, hand in hand, with our Father in heaven. We are celebrating your freedom. Now it is your turn to celebrate your rebirth. I love you. Never forget that I am by your side."

Archangel Raphael.

Energy Cleansing Bath

There is a strong energy present—an energy of liberation. Archangel Michael wants to greet you. He says he is here to guide you and that you are divinely adored and liberated.

For the bath, you will need:

- Colorful flowers
- White and red carnations
- Bay leaves
- Cinnamon
- Vanilla
- Rosemary

Boil everything except the flowers. Once the bay leaves, cinnamon, vanilla, and rosemary have boiled for 30 minutes, turn off the heat. Then add the colorful flowers and the white and red carnations, cover the pot, and wait for this infusion to reach a comfortable temperature for you before using it to bathe.

If you have the fortune of having a bathtub, you can pour this infusion into it, immerse yourself, and enjoy a bath. You can stay in the tub for as long as you want until the water cools down.

Remember that you do not towel dry after these baths. Simply dry your intimate areas, like your underarms, and wrap a towel around your head to prevent dripping. For the rest of your body, allow it to absorb all the energy and healing work from this bath.

Reminder: For every exercise, we continue to open the sacred space using the prayer we learned from the beginning of this book. So, when you perform this cleansing bath, it's also essential to open your sacred space.

With this, we close the first part of the third section of this book. Please, when you practice each of the exercises, allow yourself at least one week to observe the results. Below, I will provide you with some worksheets where you can record how you feel after completing this third part of the book within yourself.

Impact on Your Life

How do you believe the exercises and meditations from this section have impacted your life and emotional healing?

Commitments and Actions

What actions and commitments are you willing to take to maintain this healing in your daily life?

General Reflection on the Healing Process

Personal Progress Evaluation

How do you feel after working through the different sections of this book?

Key Discoveries

What were the most significant discoveries you made about yourself during this process?

Challenges Faced

What were the biggest challenges you faced during your healing process? How did you overcome them?

Notable Changes

What changes have you noticed in your emotional, physical, and spiritual life since you began this healing journey?

Integration of Tools and Exercises

Most Effective Tools

Which tools or exercises from the book did you find most effective, and why?

Application of the Tools

How do you plan to continue using these tools and exercises in your daily life?

Maintaining Progress

What strategies will you implement to maintain and continue your progress in the future?

Spiritual Connection

How has your spiritual connection changed during this process? What practices have helped you strengthen it?

Spiritual Guidance and Support

Which spiritual guides, angels, or entities do you feel have supported you during this journey? How will you communicate with them in the future?

Gratitude

Take a moment to express your gratitude for the people, experiences, and spiritual entities that have supported you on this path.

Personal Acknowledgment

Acknowledge yourself for the courage, dedication, and self-love you have shown in embarking on this healing journey.

Author's Final Note

Dear Reader,

Congratulations on making it this far. You have done deep and meaningful work on your path to healing and liberation. I hope the tools, exercises, and meditations in this book have been of great help to you, and that you continue to apply them in your daily life.

Always remember that healing is an ongoing process, and every step you take brings you closer to a life filled with peace, love, and abundance. Move forward with courage and determination, knowing that you are not alone on this journey. The angels, your spiritual guides, and the universe are always with you, supporting you every step of the way.

With love and gratitude,
Sangeeta Kalyan Kaur

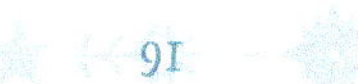

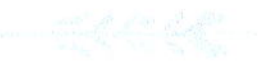

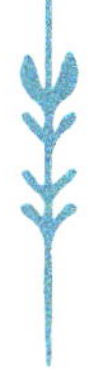

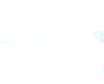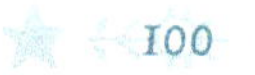

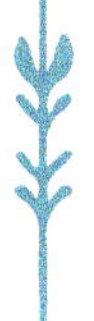

www.ingramcontent.com/pod-product-compliance
Lightning Source LLC
Chambersburg PA
CBHW051754250726
48659CB00001B/405